Sameh Mezri
Sameh Sayhi

IMPACT OF ALLERGIC RHINITIS ON SEROUS OTITIS IN CHILDREN

Sameh Mezri
Sameh Sayhi

IMPACT OF ALLERGIC RHINITIS ON SEROUS OTITIS IN CHILDREN

ScienciaScripts

Imprint

Any brand names and product names mentioned in this book are subject to trademark, brand or patent protection and are trademarks or registered trademarks of their respective holders. The use of brand names, product names, common names, trade names, product descriptions etc. even without a particular marking in this work is in no way to be construed to mean that such names may be regarded as unrestricted in respect of trademark and brand protection legislation and could thus be used by anyone.

Cover image: www.ingimage.com

This book is a translation from the original published under ISBN 978-620-6-71605-1.

Publisher:
Sciencia Scripts
is a trademark of
Dodo Books Indian Ocean Ltd. and OmniScriptum S.R.L publishing group

120 High Road, East Finchley, London, N2 9ED, United Kingdom
Str. Armeneasca 28/1, office 1, Chisinau MD-2012, Republic of Moldova, Europe
Printed at: see last page
ISBN: 978-620-7-91019-9

TABLE OF CONTENTS

INTRODUCTION

Seromucosal otitis (SMO) is defined as the presence of an aseptic serous effusion in the middle ear cavities without evidence of acute infection [1].

It is a frequent pathology in the paediatric population, with a prevalence at school age of between 15 and 20% [2], and is the leading cause of hearing loss in children. Although it may resolve spontaneously or with medical treatment, its persistence can have repercussions on the acquisition of language and speech, with major impacts on the quality of life of the child and their families. The pathogenesis of OSM is multifactorial. Allergy, and in particular allergic rhinitis, has been identified as an independent risk factor for OSM. According to the literature, the prevalence of allergic rhinitis in patients with OSM can be as high as 80% [3].

Allergic rhinitis is an IgE-mediated inflammation of the nose associated with typical symptoms such as nasal pruritus, sneezing, nasal obstruction and rhinorrhoea. It causes eustachian tube dysfunction and immune dysregulation, leading to inflammation of the middle ear cavities. Early diagnosis and adequate therapeutic control of this pathology is necessary in the management of OSM, particularly in the paediatric population. However, few studies have looked at the influence of allergic rhinitis on the therapeutic management of seromucous otitis, particularly surgery. The aim of our study was to describe the impact of allergic rhinitis on clinical, therapeutic and audiometric outcomes in children undergoing surgery for seromucous otitis.

METHODS

1. Type of study:

We conducted a retrospective descriptive study of the records of patients operated on for seromucous otitis in the Department of Otolaryngology (ENT) and Head and Neck Surgery at the Tunis Military Hospital, during the period from 2014 to 2021.

2. Population of the study:

2.1. Inclusion criteria :

Children were included in this study:

• school-age children (aged between five and nine).

• who had undergone surgery for seromucous otitis, with placement of a trans-tympanic airway (TTA), during the study period.

• with a minimum postoperative follow-up of 12 months.

• having at least two post-operative audiometric checks with ATT in place: the first between one and three months after surgery and the second at six months.

• with an audiometric check after removal of the ATT.

2.2. Non inclusion criteria:

Children were not included:

• Having of pathologies otological associated which maydistort the interpretation of results (additional conductive hearing loss).

• who were referred for surgery but failed to attend their appointments.

2.3. Exclusion criteria :

Children were excluded from this study:

• who have not had a clinical check-up (less than 12 months follow-up) and/or postoperative audiometry.

• aged over nine years at the time of surgery.

• with additional pathology such as congenital malformations (such as cleft palate, ossicular aplasia, trisomy 21) and untreated gastro-oesophageal reflux disease (GERD) at the time of surgery.

3. Methods:

3.1.Collection of data:

Data were collected from outpatient consultation forms, medical records and operative reports.

All these data were recorded on a pre-established information sheet specific to each patient (Appendix 1).

For each patient, we specified:

► Data from the interview:

- Gender, age

- Personal history

- Functional symptomatology (otological signs, rhinological signs and impact on language, speech and schooling)
► Physical examination data:

- General examination

- Ear, nose and throat examination (otoscopic, rhinological and oropharyngeal examination)
► Results of paraclinical investigations:

- Audiometric tests: impedencemetry, tonal audiometry, auditory evoked potentials (AEP).

- Speech and language assessment

- Allergological work-up: Total immunoglobulin E (IgE) assay, multi-allergy test (Phadiatop), allergen skin test (TCA): prick test, monospecific IgE test (CLA to tyre allergens).
► Medical treatment:

For each patient, the drugs received, their dosage, the number of doses taken and the duration of treatment were recorded.
► Surgical treatment:

For each child, the indication for ATT insertion, the type of ATT inserted, the surgeries associated with the same operation and the immediate post-operative follow-up were specified.

► Post-operative evolution:

Clinical and audiometric changes were recorded during the insertion of the ATT (at one to three months and at six months) and after its removal.

► Duration of follow-up and cases of recurrence. We divided the patients into two groups:

- Group 1: children with OSM associated with allergic rhinitis (AR)

- Group 2: children with OSM without AR

For each group, we compared the age of the OSM, the effect of medical treatment, pre- and post-operative clinical data, and pre- and post-operative audiometry (ATT in place and after removal).

3.2. Definitions:

• The diagnosis of OSM was based on the clinical appearance on otoscopy (dull, bluish eardrum or retrotympanic bullae) and the tympanometry result (type B or C curve).

• Allergic rhinitis was defined by the presence of favourable functional and clinical signs (nasal obstruction, sneezing, nasal pruritus, rhinorrhoea) associated with at least one positive paraclinical test (prick test, specific IgE assay).

• Allergic rhinitis has been classified according to the ARIA (Allergic Rhinitis and its Impact on Asthma) classification of allergic rhinitis in its latest 2017 update (Appendix 2) in:

✓ Intermittent or persistent, depending on the duration of symptoms:

- Intermittent RA when symptoms are present for less than four weeks and less than 4 days a week.

- Persistent RA when symptoms are present for more than four weeks and more than 4 days a week.

✓ Mild or moderate to severe, depending on the intensity of the symptoms and their impact on the child's sleep and quality of life:

- Slight: does not meet the definition of moderate/severe

- Moderate to severe: meets one or more of the following criteria: sleep disturbance/impaired school performance/impairment of school performance/impairment of school performance/impairment of school performance/impairment of school performance/impairment of school performance.

Impairment of daily activities and leisure activities/ bothersome symptoms.

• Recurrent acute otitis media (AOM): number of episodes of AOM greater than or equal to three over a period of 6 months or four over a period of one year [3].

• Atopy: is defined as a genetic predisposition to produce specific IgE antibodies against environmental allergens [3].

• Sensitisation: is defined by the production of IgE antibodies specific to one or more allergens [3].

• Allergy: is the presence of symptoms and signs immediately after exposure to the sensitising allergen [3].

• Recovery was defined as a subjective improvement in hearing associated with an improvement in audiometric threshold.

• Early otorrhoea: occurring during the first month postoperatively [4].

• Secondary otorrhoea: occurring after the first postoperative month [4].

3.3. Parameters audiometric:

• Impedencemetry: used to plot the tympano-ossicular compliance curve (tympanogram) (Appendix 3):

- Type A curve: centred curve with a narrow peak corresponding to normal compliance of the tympano-ossicular system.

- Type B curve: a flat curve indicating reduced tympanic mobility due to the presence of a retro-tympanic effusion.

- Type C curve: shift of the curve towards negative pressures, indicating tubal dysfunction.

• Pure tone audiometry:

For each patient, the threshold in decibels (dB) for air conduction (AC) and bone conduction (BC) was recorded for the frequencies 500, 1000, 2000 and 4000 Hz.

The average hearing threshold in CA dB was calculated using this formula:

(threshold at 500 Hz + threshold at 1000 Hz + threshold at 2000 Hz) / 3 The functional result was assessed by comparing the hearing thresholds of the pre- and post-treatment tone audiograms, thus calculating the average hearing gain for each ear.

3.4. allergological parameters:

• Total IgE levels: measured using the chemiluminescence method. A level is considered high when it exceeds 90 IU/ml.

• Multi-allergy test (Phadiatop): was carried out using the chemiluminescence technique. It included the following allergens: Dermatophagoides, amboisia, plantain, common foxtail, cat (epithelium), dog (scales), Penicillium notatum, Alternaria tenuis, couch grass, timothy grass.

• Identification of the allergen: two methods were used: the prick test and the monospecific specific IgE test:

✓ The prick test: Only pneumallergens were tested: house dust mites: Dermatophagoides Pteronyssinus (DP) and Dermatophagoides Farinae (DF).

12 grasses/ 4 cereals/ latex/ cat hair/ cockroach/ mixed feathers/ pellitory/ 5 grasses/ cypress/ olive tree/ alteria.

The test was considered positive when the negative control was negative, the positive control was positive and the diameter of the papule was greater than 3 mm, or when the diameter was greater than half the diameter of the positive control [5]. A positive prick test indicates sensitisation to this allergen.

■ Specific IgE monospecific test: CLA 30 pneumallergens: The

Specific IgE was measured using the chemiluminescence technique. Eight families of allergens were tested: tree pollens, grass pollens, herbaceous pollens, animal dander, moulds, latex, insects and house dust mites, including 30 allergens. This test was considered positive for an allergen when its IgE concentration exceeded 0.7 IU/ml.

4. Analysis statistics:

The data were entered and analysed using IBM SPSS Statistics 25.0 software. Absolute frequencies and relative frequencies (percentages) were calculated for categorical variables. For quantitative variables, means and standard deviations, medians and inter-quartile ranges were calculated.

5. Search bibliography:

The bibliography was entered using Zotero software. The databases consulted were Pubmed and Science direct, as well as the library of the Faculty of Medicine in Tunis. The keywords used in French and English were:

- Rhinite allergique / Allergic rhinitis

- Otitis media with effusion / Seromucous otitis

- Traitement / Treatment

- Evolution / Evolution

- Audiometry / Audiometry

6. Ethical considerations and conflicts of interest:

Given its retrospective nature, this study was not subject to prior consent from the patients included. Confidentiality of medical records was respected during data collection and analysis. We declare that there were no conflicts of interest in the preparation of this study.

1. Epidemiological study :

1.1. Frequency:

During the period of our study (2014-2021), we identified 60 school-age children treated for seromucosal otitis requiring trans-tympanic aeration, a frequency of 7.5/year. Allergic rhinitis was diagnosed in 26 children. Its prevalence in our series was 43%.

1.2. Breakdown by gender:

Our study included 32 boys and 28 girls, giving a sex ratio of 1.14.

1.3. Breakdown by age:

The average age of our population was 6.5 years [5-9 years]. We noted a peak at the age of 6. Sixty-five per cent of these children were under 8 years of age.

2. Study clinical:

2.1. History of pathological :

Forty-three per cent of the children had a pathological history (Table I).

Table I: Distribution of children according to pathological history.

Pathological history	Workforce	Percentage (%)
Allergic asthma	4	7
Recurrent sore throat	12	20
Acute recurrent otitis media	14	23

2.2. Environment:

Environmental data was available in 70% of cases (N=42). Of these cases, 22 were exposed to environmental risk factors for OSM. This table summarises the various environmental risk factors to which these children are exposed (Table II).

Table II: Distribution of children according to environmental risk factors.

Environment	Workforce	Percentage (%)
Passive smoking	5	11,9
Humidity	7	16,7
Community life	12	28,6
Crèche attendance	20	47,6

2.3. Functional signs :

The functional signs reported at the time of consultation were dominated by hearing loss in both groups, noted in 83% of cases (Table III).

Table III: Distribution of children in the two groups according to functional signs.

Functional sign (%)	Group with RA		Total (%)
Hearing loss	77	88	83
Earache	38	29	33
Language delay	15	23	20
School delay	11	19	17
Nasal pruritus	100	0	43
Nasal obstruction	100	6	78
Sneezing	100	0	43
Rhinorrhea	92	11	78
Nocturnal snoring	54	19	35
Mouth breathing	15	11	13

In the OSM with AR group, 43% of children had persistent symptoms, and 23% suffered from disturbed sleep and/or an impact on their daily activities (Figure 1).

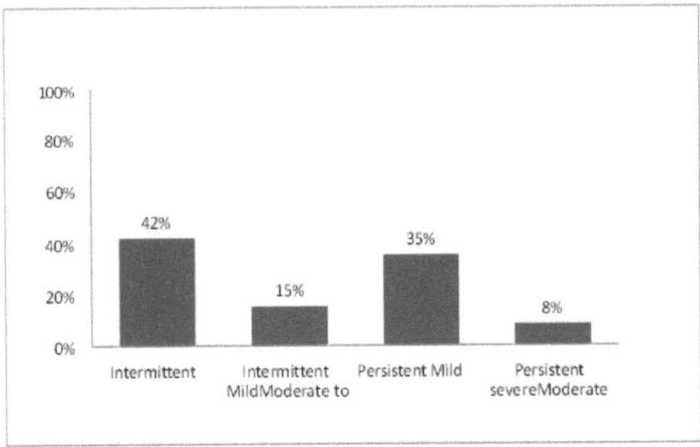

Figure 1: Distribution of children in the OSM group with AR according to the ARIA classification of their allergic rhinitis.

3.4.Seniority of l'OSM

The average follow-up time for seromucosal otitis before surgical treatment was 13 months for both groups (11 months for the OSM without RA group and 16 months for the OSM with RA group).

3.5.Examination :

3.5.1. Examination :

All the children were in good general health at the time of consultation. We were unable to calculate body mass index (BMI) due to lack of data.

3.5.2. Examination otology:

Otoscopy was consistent with bilateral OSM in all children. The eardrum was dull in 91.6% of the ears examined (Table IV).

Table IV: Distribution of children according to the result of the otoscopic examination.

Otoscopic appearance	Group without RA		Group with RA	
	OD	OG	OD	OG
Dull tympanum	32	31	24	23
Retro-tympanic bubbles	1	2	1	1
Bluish tympanum	1	0	0	0
Shrink pocket	0	1	1	2
Total	34	34	26	26

OD: right ear, **OG:** left ear

3.5.3. Rhinological examination :

Anterior rhinoscopy was normal in 43% of children. For the remainder, it revealed hypertrophy of the inferior turbinates (HCI) and clear rhinorrhoea in 43% and 20% of cases respectively (Figure 2).

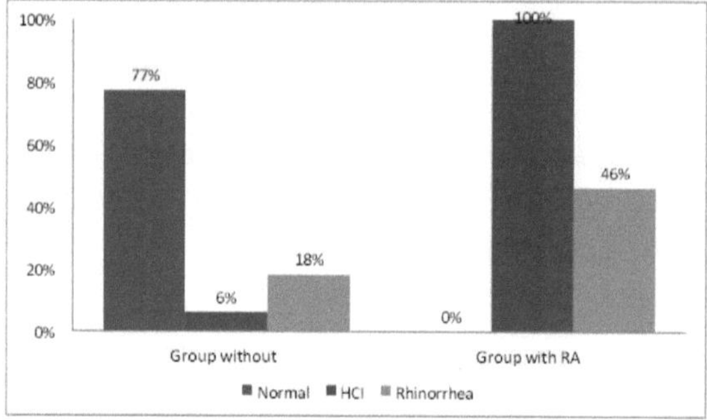

Figure 2: Distribution of children according to the result of the rhinological examination.

Nasal endoscopy, performed in 84% of cases, revealed hypertrophic adenoids in 74% of cases, 32% of which were obstructive (Figure 3).

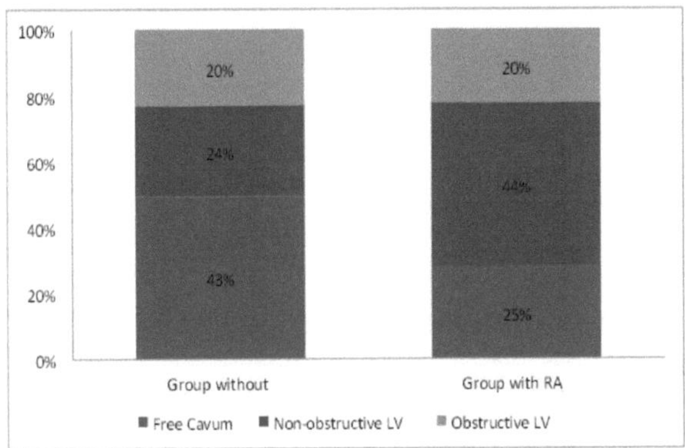

Figure 3: Distribution of children according to the result of the endoscopic examination.

3.5.4. Examination oropharyngeal:

Examination of the oropharynx revealed hypertrophic palatine tonsils (AP) in 57% of cases, 18% of which were obstructive (Figure 4).

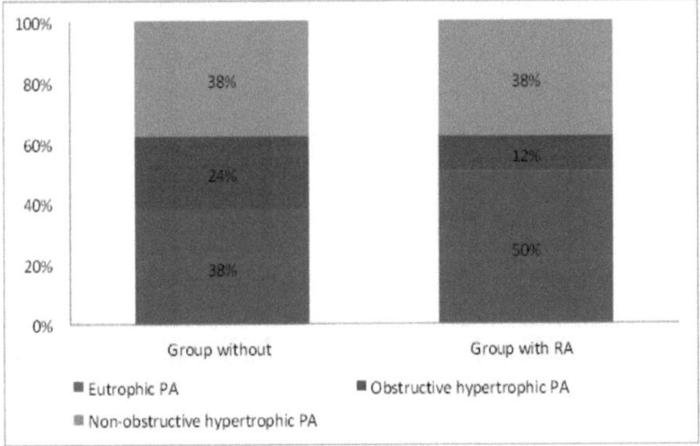

Figure 4: Distribution of children according to the result of the oropharyngeal examination.

4. Paraclinical investigations :

4.1. Initial audiometric test :

4.1.1. Impedance measurement :

Impedancemetry was performed in all our patients. The tympanogram curve was type B in 83% of cases. The remainder showed a type C curve. All children in the OSM group with AR had a type B tympanogram, while 70% of children without AR had a type B tympanogram (Figure 5).

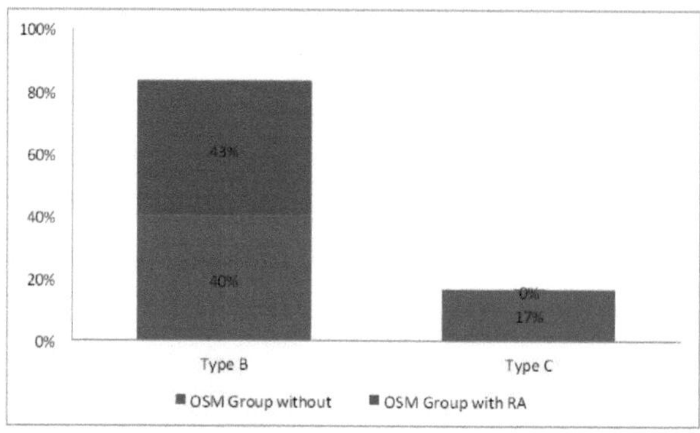

Figure 5: Distribution of children according to tympanogram result.

4.1.2. Audiometry :

Audiometry was carried out on all the children. It revealed a bilateral conductive hearing loss in all cases. The mean threshold was 42 dB [30-55 dB] for the right ear and 40 dB [28-52 dB] for the left ear (Figure 6 and Table V).

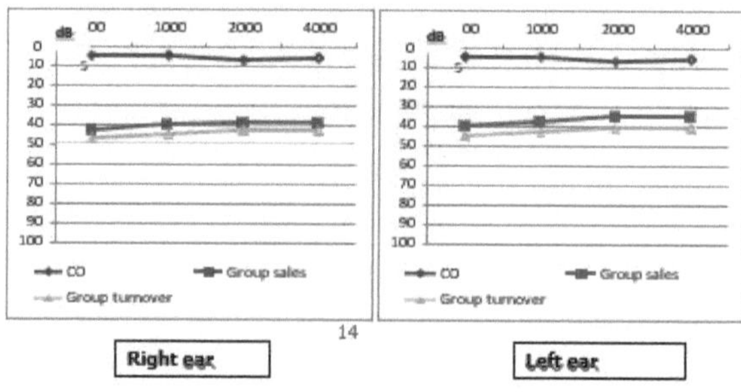

Figure 6: Average hearing threshold for children in the two groups.

Table V: Average hearing loss for children in both groups before surgical treatment.

Average hearing threshold (dB)

	Group without RA	**Group with RA**
Right ear	41 [30 - 50]	44 [35 - 55]
Left ear	38 [28 - 47]	42 [30 - 52]
Two ears	39,5	43

4.1.3. Auditory evoked potentials :

A PEA was requested for seven patients because of doubt about their hearing threshold on pure tone audiometry. The mean threshold was 44 dB [40-50] on the right and 43 dB [35-45] on the left.

4.1.4. Speech and language assessment :

A speech and language assessment was carried out on 28 children. It revealed a language delay in 15 of them. On audiometric assessment, these children had bilateral conductive hearing loss with an average threshold in the better ear of 44 dB [43-46]. These children received speech therapy.

4.2.　Allergy test :

4.2.1. Determination of total IgE antibodies :

A total IgE assay was requested in two children whose results were high (mean value of 103 IU/ml).

4.2.2. Multi-allergenic test (Phadiatop) :

This test was requested for six children. The results were positive in all cases.

4.2.3. Identification of the allergen :

4.2.3.1. The Prick test :

A pneumallergen prick test was performed on all 26 children presenting clinical symptoms suggestive of allergic rhinitis. The result was positive in 77%. Sensitivity to house dust mites was observed in 90% of positive tests (Table VI). Multiple sensitisation was noted in 90% of cases. Pollen sensitisation was found in 25% of cases (olive pollen in all cases).No food allergen tests were carried out.

Table VI: Distribution of pneumallergens.	of children according to	result of the prick test to
Raising awareness	Number of children	Percentage of tests (%)
DP+ DF	11	42
DP+ DF+ Olivier	3	11
Olivier	2	8
DP+ DF+ Alternaria	2	8
DP+ DF+ Cockroach	1	4
DP+ DF+ Cat hair	1	4
Total	20	77

4.2.3.2. Single specific IgE test :

Six children were tested for specific IgE antibodies. These children had symptoms suggestive of allergic rhinitis and a negative prick test. It revealed sensitisation to house dust mites (DP and DF) in all cases. At the end of this allergological investigation, the diagnosis of allergic rhinitis was confirmed in 26 children. House dust mites (DP+DF) were the most frequent allergens involved, found in 24 children (92%) (Figure 6).

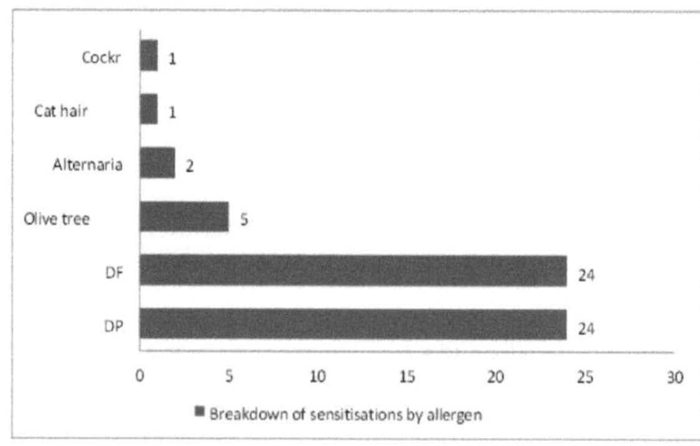

Figure 7: Breakdown of sensitisations by allergen.

5. Treatment medical:

Once the diagnosis of OSM had been made, initial medical treatment was instituted for all the children. For the group whose diagnosis of allergic rhinitis was confirmed, a specific treatment was prescribed.

Figure 7 summarises the various medical treatments administered to the two groups.

5.1. Antibiotic therapy :

Antibiotic therapy (ATB) based on amoxicillin was prescribed for 28 children (46.7%), at an average dose of 80 mg/kg/d, and for an average duration of seven days.Of these children, 68% (N=19) belonged to the OSM with RA group (Figure 7).

5.2. Oral corticosteroid therapy :

Half of the children received oral prednisolone-based corticosteroid therapy (CT) at a mean dose of 1mg/kg/d (N=30). The average number of courses was two per year. Sixty per cent of these children belonged to the OSM with RA group.

5.3. Oral antihistamine :

All children with a confirmed diagnosis of allergic rhinitis (N=26) received an oral antihistamine (HA). The most commonly used molecule was Cetirizine (Allergica@) (for 18 children), at a dose of 5mg/d for children under the age of six and 10mg/d for children aged □ six. For the rest, the drug prescribed was Desloratadine (Deslor@) at a dose of 5mg/day. The average duration of treatment was 14 months [2 - 24 months].

5.4. Treatment by nasal route :

-Nasal cleansing with saline solution

Nasal cleansing with physiological saline was prescribed for all children.

-Nasal corticosteroid therapy

Nasal corticosteroid therapy (CT) was initiated in 70% of the children (N=42). Of these children, 43.3% had allergic rhinitis (OSM group with AR). The drug used was Fluticasone (Rinosal@ , Flixonase@) at a daily dose of 50ug/d in 64.3% of cases (N=27) and Tixocortol pivalate (Pivalone 1%@) at a dose of one spray/day in the remaining cases (N=15). The average duration of treatment was 8 months [4 - 24 months].

-Blown derivatives:

Fifteen children (25%) received nasal puffed derivatives (Actisouffre).[@]

5.5.Immunotherapy allergen:

Four children received allergen immunotherapy (AIT). The allergen involved was DP+DF in three cases and olive tree in one case. The sublingual route was used in all cases. The average duration was four years [3-5 years].

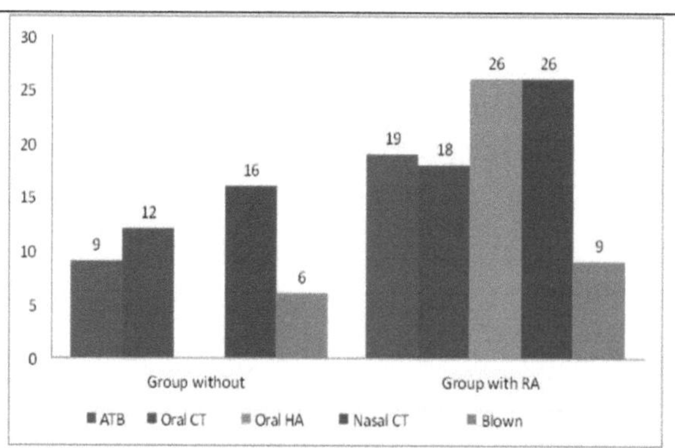

Figure 8: Breakdown of the different medical treatments administered for the two groups.

6. Treatment surgical:

When medical treatment failed to improve, all the children were fitted with a trans-tympanic airway (TTA).

6.1. Indications for treatment surgery:

In all cases, a hearing threshold of more than 30 dB was the reason for fitting the ATT, and in 15 cases this was associated with a language impairment.

6.2. Surgical procedure

The surgical procedure was performed under general anaesthetic in all cases. The ATT used was a Teflon "T"-shaped ATT. Ninety per cent of the children had bilateral ATT placement. Sixteen children with obstructive adenoids underwent adenoidectomy at the same time, and ten had their palatine tonsils removed.No intraoperative incidents were reported.

6.3.Surgery immediately:

All the children underwent at least six hours of postoperative monitoring. No complications were noted in the immediate postoperative period. All patients were discharged the same day.

7. Post-surgical evolution of seromucous otitis :

7.1.Check-up at one to three months post operation:

7.1.1. Results

A subjective improvement in hearing was reported in all children.At follow-up otoscopy, the ATT was in place in all cases. Otorrhea was observed in nine cases, prompting the prescription of antibiotic ear drops for an average of seven days. Of these children, seven were in the OSM with RA group (77.8%). In the case of one child, whose otorrhoea persisted, oral antibiotic therapy was prescribed and the otorrhoea subsided after seven days of treatment.

7.1.2. Results audiometric:

An improvement in audiometric threshold was noted in all children. The mean audiometric threshold was 22 dB on the right [15 - 27 dB] and 20 dB on the left [13 - 25 dB], giving a mean gain of 20 dB. This gain was higher for the OSM group without RA (21.5 dB), compared with 18 dB for the group with RA (Table VII, Figure 8).

Table VII: Average hearing gain one to three months after trans-tympanic aerator insertion in both ears and for both groups.

Average gain (dB)	OSM Group without RA	OSM Group with RA
Right ear	19 [14 - 22]	19 [14 - 24]
Left ear	20 [16 - 24]	17 [12 - 21]
Two sides	21,5 [15 - 23]	18 [13 - 22,5]

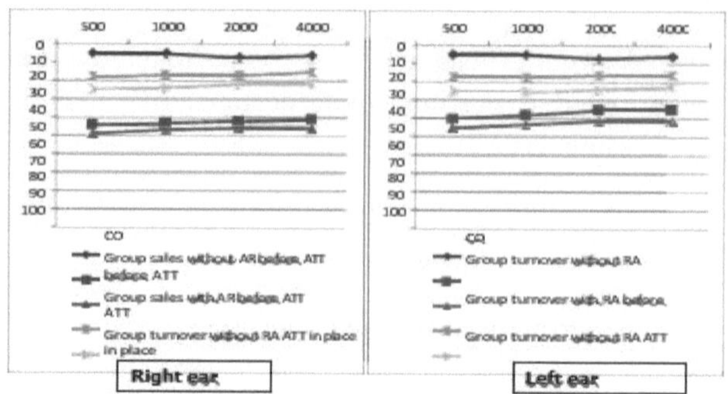

Figure 9: Mean pure-tone audiometry before the insertion of the ATT and at one to three months afterwards for children in both groups.

7.2. Six-month check-up post operation:

7.2.1. Results

A stable improvement in clinical symptoms was noted in all children.At follow-up otoscopy, the ATT was in place in all cases. There were no cases of ATT migration.Otorrhea was detected in ten cases, eight of which were in the OSM with RA group (80%). Of these cases, seven were concomitant with an episode of rhinitis and the other three with swimming. Local antibiotic therapy was administered to all these children, with improvement after an average of eight days' treatment.

7.2.2. Results audiometric:

The mean audiometric threshold was 24 dB on the right [20 - 30 dB] and 23 dB on the left [15 - 28 dB], giving a mean gain of 17.5 dB. This gain was higher for the OSM group without RA (18.5 dB), compared with 16 dB for the group with RA (Table VIII, Figure 9).

Table VIII: Average hearing gain at six months after trans-tympanic aerator insertion in both ears and for both groups.

Average gain (dB)	OSM Group without RA	OSM Group with RA
Right ear	20 [18 - 27]	17 [14 - 22]
Left ear	17 [15 - 25]	15 [13 - 20]
Two sides	18,5 [16,5- 26]	16 [13,5 - 21]

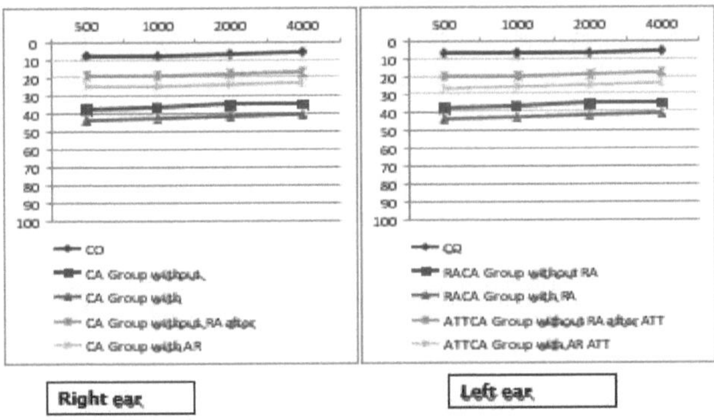

Figure 10: Mean pure-tone audiometry before and 6 months after the insertion of the TTE for both groups.

7.3. Check after removal of :

7.3.1. Installation time of l'ATT:

The average duration of the ATT was 13 months [8-18 months]. Spontaneous removal of the ATT was noted in ten children, six of whom were in the OSM with RA group (60%). The average delay was 9 months [8-12 months]. In the other cases, removal took place after an average of 14 months [10-18 months].

7.3.2. Results

The improvement in hearing was stable in 86% of cases.On otoscopy, the eardrum returned to its normal appearance in 81.7% of cases. A tympanic perforation following removal of the ATT was observed in one child, which healed completely after six months.

7.3.3. Results audiometric:

The mean audiometric threshold after removal of the ATT in both ears was 22.5 dB [15 - 29 dB]. For the OSM group without RA, this threshold was 19 dB, unlike that of the group with RA, which was 27 dB. The mean hearing gain in both ears was 18.5 dB [15-27 dB] (Table IX, Figure 10).

Table IX: Average hearing gain after removal of the trans-tympanic aerator in both ears and for both groups.

Average gain (dB)	OSM Group without RA	OSM Group with RA
Right ear	21 [18 - 25]	17 [14 - 24]
Left ear	20 [16 - 27]	15 [13 - 26]
Two sides	20,5[17- 26]	16 [13,5 - 25]

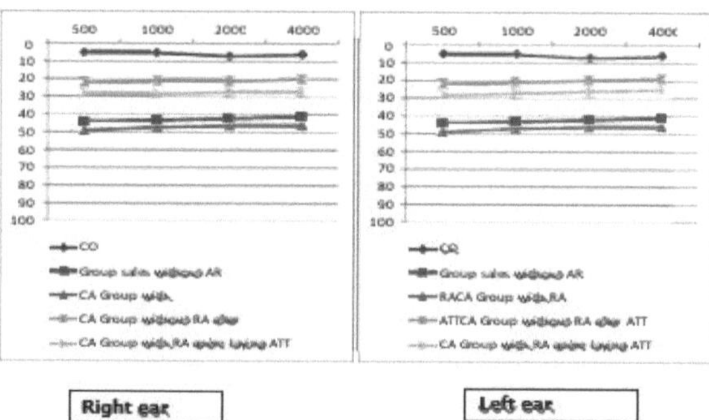

Figure 11: Mean pure-tone audiometry before and after the insertion of the ATT for children in both groups.

7.3.4. Recurrence of seromucous otitis :

OSM recurrence was observed in four children. The average delay was 14 months after removal of the TSA, with extremes ranging from 12 to 24 months. Three of these children belonged to the group with associated allergic rhinitis. These children received medical treatment based on courses of corticosteroids. Clinical and audiometric improvement was observed in two patients. The other two were lost to follow-up.

7.3.5. Post-operative setback

The mean follow-up time after the introduction of ATT was 17 months, with extremes ranging from 12 to 39 months. A total of 32% of children developed otorrhoea postoperatively, 25% of whom were in the OSM with RA group, 17% had early expulsion of the ATT and 2% had residual perforation. Recurrence of OSM after removal of the ATT was observed in 7% of children, 5% of whom were in the OSM with RA group (Figure 11).

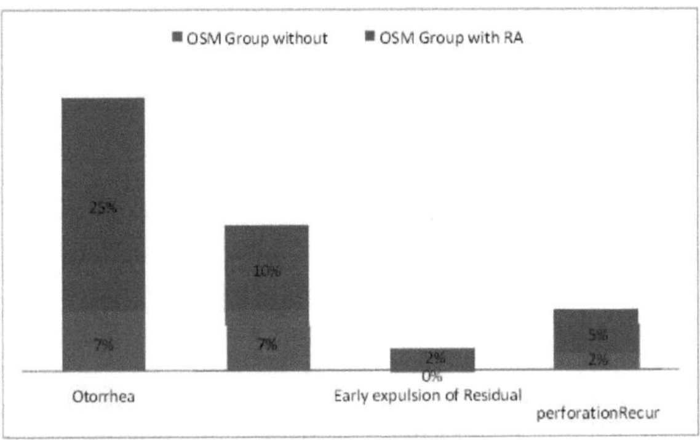

Figure 12: Distribution of children in the two groups according to complications arising after the insertion of the ATT.

DISCUSSION

1. The main results of our study:

The aim of our study was to describe the impact of allergic rhinitis on clinical, therapeutic and audiometric outcomes in children undergoing surgery for seromucous otitis.To this end, we conducted a monocentric retrospective study of the records of children treated surgically for seromucous otitis at the Department of Otolaryngology and Head and Neck Surgery of the Tunis Military Hospital, during the period from 2014 to 2021.School-age children (aged between 5 and 9 years) who had undergone surgery for an OSM, with an ATT fitted, during the study period were included. We required a minimum postoperative follow-up of 12 months and a postoperative audiometric check with the ATT in place between one and three months after surgery, then at six months and an audiometric check after its removal. We divided the children into two groups: a group with OSM associated with allergic rhinitis and a group with OSM without allergic rhinitis.Our series included 60 children, representing a frequency of 7.5 cases per year. The mean age was 6.5 years. The sex ratio was 1.14. Pathological history was dominated by recurrent AOM found in 23% of cases. Crèche attendance was the most common environmental factor. Functional otological signs were dominated by hypoacusis (83%) and rhinological signs dominated by nasal obstruction and rhinorrhoea (78% each). OSM was bilateral in all children. The eardrum was dull in 91.6% of the ears examined.Children in the OSM with AR group were more likely to have a type B tympanogram (100% compared with 70% for the group without AR). The mean hearing threshold was higher for the OSM with AR group (43 dB compared with 39.5 dB for the other group). All children with symptoms of allergic rhinitis underwent an allergological assessment. On completion of this work-up, the diagnosis of allergic rhinitis was confirmed in 26 children (OSM group with AR). The prevalence of AR in our series was 43.3%. House dust mites (DP+DF) were the most frequent allergens involved, found in 92.3% of these children. A comparison of the medical treatments received by the two groups showed a higher frequency of prescription of oral corticosteroids and antibiotics in the children in the OSM with AR group. Subjective improvement in hearing after ATT was reported i n all children. The mean hearing gain at three and six months after ATT was lower in the OSM with AR group (18 dB vs. 21.5 dB at three months and 16 dB vs. 18.5 dB at six months for the other group). The average duration of t h e ATT was 13 months [8-18 months]. After removal of the ATT, the mean hearing threshold was 19 dB for the OSM without RA group and 27 dB for the OSM with RA group.Postoperatively, 32% of children developed otorrhea (25% in the OSM with RA group and 7% in the no RA group), 17% had early expulsion of the ATT and 2% had residual perforation. Recurrence of OSM after removal of the ATT was observed in 7% of children, 5% of whom were in the OSM with RA group. The average postoperative follow-up was 17 months.

2. Strengths and limitations of our study:

► The retrospective nature of the study: we conducted a retrospective, descriptive, longitudinal study, which, like any retrospective study, included bias :

- Information bias: data was collected uniformly using a pre-established digital form. Some data could not be collected from all patients.

- Migration bias: it is possible that some patients would have continued their treatment in other hospitals. As a result, certain complications or recurrences may not have been recorded.

- The patients were treated by different doctors with different therapeutic attitudes.

- Patient follow-up during 2020 and 2021 was not optimal given the SARS COVID19 epidemic. Some patients did not attend their follow-up appointments.

► Post-operative follow-up:

A significant number of cases were excluded, given the lack of compliance in the post-operative checks.

The duration of follow-up was not the same for all patients. It was short for some patients in order to detect recurrence.

► The sample: the total number of patients in the study was insufficient for a statistical study.

► Scope of the study: the duration of the study enabled us to evaluate the effectiveness of the ATT and to compare it between the two groups.

3. Study compared with data in the literature:

3.1. Epidemiological study :

3.1.1. Frequency:

3.1.1.1. Prevalence of seromucous otitis in children with allergic rhinitis:

The prevalence of OSM in the school-age paediatric population has been estimated at 20%. In a study by Passali et al, comparing two groups of children: one with AR and one without, the authors found that 7.5% of the AR group had OSM, compared with 1.6% of the non-AR group [6]. According to other authors, this prevalence may exceed 40%, underlining the role of allergy in the genesis of OSM [7]. Several mechanisms have been proposed to explain the role of allergy in the development of OSM: the inflammatory reaction and obstruction of the eustachian tube orifice, the Th2-mediated immune response in the middle ear and the aspiration of bacteria-laden allergic nasopharyngeal secretions into the middle ear cavity [8]. These mechanisms explain the high prevalence of OSM in allergic patients.

3.1.1.2. Prevalence of allergic rhinitis in children with seromucous otitis:

The incidence of allergic rhinitis in the paediatric population has been reported to be 5-10%. Over the last few decades, this prevalence in school-age children has continued to increase, as shown by the results of the international observational study ISAAC (International Study of Asthma and Allergy in Childhood) [9]. Cheng and colleagues conducted a meta-analysis including seven case-control studies of the association between allergic rhinitis and OSM. The prevalence of allergic rhinitis was three times higher in the group of children with OSM than in the control group [10]. Several studies have shown that 40 to 50 % of children aged over three with OSM suffered from AR. For Alles et al, this prevalence may exceed 80% [11]. In our series, this prevalence was 43%.

3.1.2. Age and gender:

According to the literature, the prevalence of OSM was highest in children aged between four and eight. It tends to decrease with age [12]. In a cross-sectional study involving 1,488 school-age children, Al-Humaid et al studied the risk factors for the development of OSM, particularly those relating to age. They found a statistically significant correlation between OSM and age under eight years (OR=5.052) [13]. In our study, 65% of children with persistent OSM were under the age of eight. The variability of the sex ratio found in the series cannot confirm a predominance of sex in children with OSM (Table X).

Table X: Comparison of average age and sex ratio with the literature.

StudyNumber of cases Mean age Sex ratio

Norhafizah et al [12]	130	8	1,06
Martines et al [7]	40	5,5	0,4
Our study	60	6,5	1,14

3.1.3. Medical and surgical history :

Saim et al, studied the medical risk factors for OSM in a study including 1097 children. A history of AOM, allergic rhinitis, recurrent angina and craniofacial anomalies were statistically associated with a higher risk of OSM [14]. In our series, in addition to AR, 23.3% of children had recurrent AOM, 20% had recurrent tonsillitis and 7% had allergic asthma.

3.1.4. Factors :

3.1.4.1. Environmental risk factors for seromucous otitis :

Saim et al, highlighted the non-medical risk factors influencing the onset of OSM. These included, in addition to age, family size, history of OSM in siblings, short duration or absence of breastfeeding and passive smoking [14]. Norhafizah et al also found a statistically significant relationship between family size of four or more and the development of persistent OSM [12].

3.1.4.2. Environmental risk factors for allergic rhinitis :

In a 2009 cross-sectional Tunisian study of 200 children,

Statistical analysis of the various risk factors for sensitisation concluded that these factors, in addition to family and personal atopy, were: short duration of breastfeeding and dampness of the home. On the other hand, no correlation was found for passive smoking, rural or urban living environment, age of dietary diversification and infections at an early age [15]. The presence of environmental factors common to OSM and RA reinforces the relationship between these two conditions.

3.2. Study clinical:

3.2.1. Functional signs of seromucous otitis and rhinitis allergic:

In the series by Norhafizah et al, hearing loss was the most common functional complaint. is common in children with persistent OSM, reported in 81.7% of cases, followed by otalgia in 16.9% [12]. In our series, 83% of children complained of hearing loss and 33% of otalgia. Experts have developed a score to help screen for allergic rhinitis: Score For Allergic Rhinitis (SFAR). This is a quantitative score ranging from 0 to 16 and encompassing eight characteristics of AR. A SFAR value greater than or equal to seven allowed satisfactory discrimination between patients with and without AR (Appendix 4).Umapathy et al, evaluated the association between symptoms in favour of OSM and those in favour of RA. They questioned 332 school-age children using a questionnaire that included otological and nasal symptoms. A statistically significant correlation was observed between symptoms suggestive of OSM and those suggestive of AR (P=0.0000) [16]. In our study, 43% of children with otological symptoms of OSM had a rhinological complaint suggestive of AR. These findings underline the importance of looking for otological symptoms in any child with AR, and for nasal symptoms in any case of OSM.

3.2.2. Classification of rhinitis allergic:

Classically, AR was divided into seasonal, perennial or mixed AR [17]. The latest update of the ARIA (Allergic Rhinitis and its Impact on Asthma) working group classifies AR according to whether it is intermittent or persistent, and whether it is mild or moderate to severe (Appendix 2). According to the study by Norhafizah et al, 63.2% of children with OSM and AR had persistent AR, the majority (33.8%) of which was of moderate to severe intensity [12]. This figure was different from that found in our study: 43% of children suffered from persistent symptoms (Table XI).

Table XI: Comparison of the classification of allergic rhinitis with the literature.

Classification of Light	Intermittent RA	Intermittent moderate to severe	Slightly persistent	Persistent moderate to severe
Norhafizah et al	13,2%	25%	29,4%	33,8%
Passali et al [6]	19%	22%	18%	41%
Our study	42%	15%	35%	8%

3.3. Paraclinical investigations

3.3.1. Investigations :

3.3.1.1. Impedencemetry:

This technique studies the compliance of the tympano-ossicular system by modifying the air pressure in the external auditory canal [1]. A flat type B curve is suggestive of a retro-tympanic effusion, with a sensitivity of 89% and a specificity of 75%. It confirms the diagnosis of OSM [18]. Martines et al, studied the tympanometry results in two groups of school-age children suffering from OSM: atopic and non-atopic children. They found that 79% of atopic children had a type B tympanogram and 21% a type C tympanogram, while 56% of non-atopic children had a type B tympanogram and 44% a type C tympanogram [7]. Thus, atopic children are more likely to have a flat tympanometry curve. They also found that atopic children are more likely to develop bilateral OSM [7]. Similarly, in our study, children with AR were more likely to have a type B tympanogram than the group without AR (100% versus 70%).

3.3.1.2. Audiometry :

Hearing loss in OSM ranges from zero dB to 55 dB. In 20% of cases, children with OSM have an average hearing threshold greater than 35 dB, and 5-10% have a threshold of 40-50 dB [19]. The study by Martinez et al, noted that 1.47% of children had a hearing loss exceeding 50dB and that all of these children suffered from associated AR [7]. Norhafizah et al, analysed the hearing threshold in two groups of children with OSM: one group with associated AR and the other without. They found a significant difference between these two groups and concluded that OSM children with AR had a significantly higher hearing threshold than children without AR [12]. Also, the study by Martines et al found a higher air conduction threshold for the frequencies 500 Hz to 4000 Hz in the group of atopic children compared with a group of non-atopic children (31.97 dB compared with 29.8 dB) [7]. The results of our study were consistent with the literature. The OSM with AR group showed a higher hearing threshold than the OSM without AR group (43 dB vs. 39.5 dB). Allergic rhinitis is therefore a factor that worsens hearing in children with OSM. Early diagnosis and effective treatment in this population could prevent the repercussions of OSM on children's hearing loss.

3.3.2. Investigations allergology:

3.3.2.1. Determination of total IgE :

Total IgE concentration is elevated in 30-40% of patients with allergic rhinitis but may be elevated in patients with other non-allergic conditions, making this parameter unreliable for the diagnosis of allergic rhinitis [20]. Sharifian et al assessed serum IgE levels in two groups of children: a group with OSM and a control group. They found elevated serum IgE levels in 29.7% of the OSM group and 14.5% of the control group. However, no significant difference was observed between the two groups [16].

3.3.2.2. Multi- allergen tests:

Multi-allergen screening tests correspond to assay techniques that look for serum IgE antibodies to different allergens fixed on the same support. Bchir et al studied the correlation between allergen tests. They found a correlation between the Phadiatop and the prick test of 92% for children. Phadiatop had a specificity of 100%, a sensitivity of 92% and an efficacy of 96% for children [21]. It can be used in patients with little suspicion of allergic rhinitis in order to rule out this diagnosis [21]. In our series, Phadiatop was requested in six children, and the results were positive in all cases.

3.3.2.3. Identification of the allergen:

a. Skin test allergenic:

Immediate-read skin tests (prick tests) are the first stage in allergological diagnosis. A cross-sectional Tunisian study conducted in 2009 included 200 children for whom a skin test to 12 common pneumallergens was performed. The prevalence of sensitisation to pneumallergens was 14%. House dust mites (DP and/or DF) were the allergens implicated in the majority of cases (96.4% of cases) [15]. Another Tunisian study carried out in 2015 examined the results of the pneumallergen prick test performed on 1,830 children. The most common pneumallergens found were house dust mites (72.1%), followed by animal dander (35.7%) and pollens (34.9%). Polysensitisation to at least two different families of pneumallergens was found in 51.4% of children [22].In our series, 90% of positive skin tests showed sensitisation to house dust mites. Multiple sensitisation was also observed in 90% of cases.

b. Determination of specific IgE antibodies :

Because of its cost, the determination of specific serum IgE is only justified as a first-line test when skin tests are not feasible (extensive dermatosis) or cannot be interpreted. However, it is still useful when there is a discrepancy between the clinically suspected allergen and the results of skin tests, or when you want to investigate sensitivity to an allergen that is not available in skin tests. It is also recommended if specific desensitisation is being considered [23]. In our series, six children in the OSM group with RA, whose skin test was negative, benefited from a specific IgE assay.

c. Nasal provocation tests :

Nasal provocation tests to allergens are useful in the diagnosis of rhinitis, when there is a discrepancy between the history, skin tests and the specific IgE assay, or when one wishes to avoid a bronchial provocation test in an asthmatic patient, for example, or in certain allergic rhinitis of occupational origin [24]. In our series, no nasal challenge test was performed.

3.4. Treatment medical:

3.4.1. The corticosteroid therapy:

Corticosteroids are commonly used in clinical practice for the treatment of OSM, despite guidelines advising against their use due to their long-term ineffectiveness and possible adverse effects [1]. Simpson et al, reviewed the use of oral and topical corticosteroids in children with OSM. Their meta-analysis included 12 studies of hearing loss caused by OSM with a total of 945 children. No benefit on resolution of OSM was found beyond one month of follow-up with oral or intra-nasal corticosteroids (used alone or with antibiotics) [25]. In our series, 50% of children received oral corticosteroids, 30% of whom had associated RA.

3.4.2. Antibiotic therapy:

Bacterial infection has long been implicated in the genesis of seromucosal otitis. However, it has been shown that the presence of a biofilm in the middle ear could probably protect the bacteria from the action of antibiotics [26]. Mandel et al, concluded that a combination of amoxicillin-clavulanic acid-based TBAs could be used temporarily to treat seromucosal otitis.   childrenDiscussion Improving symptoms before surgical treatment. Antibiotics should no longer be used routinely, given their limited benefit in relation to their cost and the emergence of resistant strains [26]. In our series, 46.7% of children received an ATB, 31.7% of whom were in the OSM with RA group. Given these results, we can assume that the presence of RA increases the use of corticosteroids and antibiotics in the management of OSM in children.

3.4.3. Antihistamines and nasal decongestants :

Several meta-analyses, systematic reviews and international consensuses have highlighted the position of antihistamines in the management of OSM. In a review of the literature, Flynn and Griffin examined 16 studies of children with OSM concerning the administration of antihistamines and/or decongestants. Their work included 1,880 participants. They found no statistical or clinical benefit for either treatment. Even so, side effects were more frequent in treated subjects than in untreated subjects [27]. Antihistamines should therefore not be used routinely in children with SMO, but only in children with an associated allergy [27].Antihistamines act on the early phase of the allergic response, the main mediator of which is histamine. Analysis of the middle ear mucosa and effusion of atopic patients with OSM shows a predominance of eosinophils and high levels of interleukin 5, which corresponds to the late phase of the allergic response. Therefore, antihistamines should have no effect on the pathophysiology of OSM [27]. In our series, antihistamines were used exclusively in children with a confirmed diagnosis of AR. In 2018, an international consensus on the management of OSM in children was reached. It recommends against the use of corticosteroids, antibiotics, decongestants or antihistamines to treat OSM due to side effects, cost issues and lack of convincing evidence of long-term efficacy [28].

3.4.4. Anti-allergenic immunotherapy :

It is now accepted that ITA is the only aetiological treatment for IgE-mediated allergic diseases such as allergic rhinitis. In addition to treating symptoms, ITA seems to have a preventive effect on the appearance of new allergen sensitisations in mono-sensitised subjects and the progression of allergic rhinitis to asthma [30].The mucous membranes of the nose and middle ear are similar. Thus, the mucosa of the middle ear is just as capable of an allergic response as the rest of the upper respiratory tract. The demonstration of Th2-type responses in the middle ears of atopic patients reinforces the hypothesis of allergic inflammation in the genesis of OSM in the atopic population [31]. In a study of 89 atopic patients with OSM, specific allergen immunotherapy completely resolved 85% of the diseased ears and significantly improved a further 5.5%. No cases of recurrence of OSM were observed in the children during 2 to 8 years of follow-up. These results support the role of allergy in the development of OSM [32].

3.5. Surgical treatment: placement of a trans- tympanic aerator:

The aim of ATT placement is to restore normal ventilation in the middle ear and drain the retro-tympanic effusion.

3.5.1. Effectiveness of trans-tympanic ventilation on hearing:

Browning et al, conducted a Cochrane review in 2010 to assess the effectiveness of ATT in controlling hearing loss due to OSM. This review included 10 randomised studies and 1728 participants. A hearing benefit was observed in t h e first 6 months after the fitting of ATT, with a mean gain of 12 dB at three months and 4 dB at 6-9 months [33]. In our study, the average gain was 15 dB at three months and 16.7 dB at six months. Similarly, Hellström et al, in their 2011 review of the literature, concluded that ATT improves hearing threshold in the first nine months after fitting [34]. However, no long-term benefit on speech and language development was demonstrated. Thus, it has been argued that the application of ATT in the treatment of OSM improves hearing thresholds as long as the aerator is in place and permeable [35].

3.5.2. Postoperative complications of trans- tympanic aerator placement:

Short- and medium-term complications of ATT are dominated by otorrhoea. Its frequency varies from 10 to 26% of cases [35]. In our study, children with with associated AR were more likely to develop otorrhoea after ATT (25% compared with 7% for children without AR).It is estimated that the frequency of premature expulsion of an ATT is 3.9% [50]. It was 10% in the OSM with RA group in our series. The incidence of residual perforations has been estimated at 3% of cases, and is correlated with the duration and number of times the ATT is inserted [35]. This figure was 2% in our study.

3.5.3. Impact of allergic rhinitis on trans- tympanic aerator placement:

In a cohort study involving 323 children, the incidence of the application of a TAA in children without a history of atopy was compared. It was found that children with allergic rhinitis in the first 12 years of life had a significantly higher incidence of TAA than non-allergic children [36]. Wang et al studied the recurrence of OSM after ATT insertion. They found a prevalence of OSM recurrence after ATT removal or extrusion of 59.6% in children with associated AR, which was higher than the overall prevalence rate of 38.7%. The prevalence of allergic rhinitis in children with a second ATT insertion was 68%, which was higher than the rate of 29% in cured children [37].

In our study, recurrence of OSM after removal of the ATT was observed in 7% of children, 5% of whom had associated AR. These results reinforce the importance of screening for and treating allergic rhinitis in the management of OSM.

CONCLUSIONS

Seromucous otitis is a common condition in the paediatric population, with a prevalence of 15-20% at school age. Allergy, and in particular allergic rhinitis, has been identified as an independent risk factor for SMO.The aim of our study was to describe the impact of allergic rhinitis on clinical, therapeutic and audiometric outcomes in children undergoing surgery for seromucous otitis. To this end, we conducted a monocentric retrospective study of the records of children treated surgically for seromucous otitis at the Department of Otolaryngology and Head and Neck Surgery of the Tunis Military Hospital, during the period from 2014 to 2021.School-age children (aged between 5 and 9 years) who had undergone surgery for an OSM, with the fitting of a trans-tympanic airway (TTA), during the study period were included. We required a minimum postoperative follow-up of 12 months and a postoperative audiometric check with the TTA in place between one and three months after surgery, then at six months and an audiometric check after its removal.We divided the children into two groups: a group with confirmed allergic rhinitis (OSM group with AR) and a group without allergic rhinitis (OSM group without AR).Our series included 60 children, representing a frequency of 7.5 cases per year. The mean age was 6.5 years. The sex ratio was 1.14. Pathological history was dominated by recurrent AOM found in 23% of cases. Crèche attendance was the most common environmental factor. Functional otological signs were dominated by hypoacusis (83%) and rhinological signs dominated by nasal obstruction and rhinorrhoea (78% each). OSM was bilateral in all children. The eardrum was dull in 91.6% of the ears examined.Children in the OSM with AR group were more likely to have a type B tympanogram (100% compared with 70% for the group without AR). The mean hearing threshold was higher for the OSM with AR group (43 dB compared with 39.5 dB for the other group).All children with symptoms of allergic rhinitis underwent an allergological assessment. At the end of this assessment, the diagnosis of allergic rhinitis was confirmed in 26 children (OSM group with AR).The prevalence of RA in our series was 43%. House dust mites (DP+DF) were the most frequent allergens involved, found in 92% of these children.A comparison of the medical treatments received by the two groups showed a higher frequency of prescription of oral corticosteroids and antibiotics in the children in the OSM with AR group. Subjective improvement in hearing after ATT was reported in all children. The mean hearing gain at three and six months after ATT was lower in the OSM with AR group (18 dB vs. 21.5 dB at three months and 16 dB vs. 18.5 dB at six months for the other group). The average duration of the ATT was 13 months [8-18 months]. After removal of the ATT, the mean hearing threshold was 19 dB for the OSM without RA group and 27 dB for the OSM with RA group.Post-operatively, 32% of children developed otorrhea (25% in the OSM with RA group and 7% in the group without RA), 17% had early expulsion of the ATT and 2% had residual perforation. Recurrence of OSM after removal of the ATT was observed in 7% of children, 5% of whom were in the OSM with RA group. The mean post-operative follow-up was 17 months.Our study shows that allergic rhinitis is an aggravating factor in hearing loss associated with OSM. It increases the need for prescription medication, particularly corticosteroids and antibiotics. ATT is less effective in reducing hearing loss in children with AR. Finally, children suffering from AR are more likely to present post-operative complications after the application of ATT and have a higher frequency of recurrence of OSM after its removal.At the end of our study and after a review of the literature, we emphasise the role of allergy in the physiology of OSM and stress the need for early detection of allergic rhinitis in children with OSM. The SFAR questionnaire should be attached to the consultation form for each child presenting with OSM.Similarly, the diagnosis of AR in children should rule out the presence of OSM by systematically examining the eardrums and assessing hearing.

REFERENCES

1. Rosenfeld RM, Shin JJ, Schwartz SR, Coggins R, Gagnon L, Hackell JM, et al. Clinical practice guideline: otitis media with effusion (update). Otolaryngol Head Neck Surg. 2016 Feb;154 Suppl 1:1-41.

2. Zielhuis GA, Rach GH, Van Den Bosch A, Van Den Broek P. The prevalence of otitis media with effusion: a critical review of the literature. Clin Otolaryngol Allied Sci. 1990 Jun;15(3):283-8.

3. Ciprandi G, Torretta S, Marseglia GL, Licari A, Chiappini E, Benazzo M, et al. Allergy and otitis media in clinical practice. Curr Allergy Asthma Rep. 2020 Jun;20(8):33.

4. Denneny JC. Ototopical agents in the treatment of the draining ear. Am J Manag Care. 2002 Oct;8 Suppl 14:353-60.

5. Heinzerling L, Mari A, Bergmann KC, Bresciani M, Burbach G, Darsow U, et al. The skin prick test - european standards. Clin Transl Allergy. 2013 Feb;3(1):3.

6. Passali D, Passali GC, Lauriello M, Romano A, Bellussi L, Passali FM. Nasal allergy and otitis media: a real correlation? Sultan Qaboos Univ Med J. 2014 Feb;14(1):59-64.

7. Martines F, Martinciglio G, Martines E, Bentivegna D. The role of atopy in otitis media with effusion among primary school children: audiological investigation. Eur Arch Otorhinolaryngol. 2010 Nov;267(11):1673-8.

8. Yeo SG, Park DC, Eun YG, Cha CI. The role of allergic rhinitis in the development of otitis media with effusion: effect on eustachian tube function. Am J Otolaryngol. 2007 May;28(3):148-52.

9. Hahm MI, Chae Y, Kwon HJ, Kim J, Ahn K, Kim WK, et al. Do newly built homes affect rhinitis in children? The ISAAC phase III study in Korea. Allergy. 2014 Apr;69(4):479-87.

10. Caffarelli C, Savini E, Giordano S, Gianlupi G, Cavagni G. Atopy in children with otitis media with effusion. Clin Exp Allergy. 1998 May;28(5):591-6.

11. Alles R, Parikh A, Hawk L, Darby Y, Romero JN, Scadding G. The prevalence of atopic disorders in children with chronic otitis media with effusion. Pediatr Allergy Immunol. 2001 Apr;12(2):102-6.

12. Norhafizah S, Salina H, Goh BS. Prevalence of allergic rhinitis in children with otitis media with effusion. Eur Ann Allergy Clin Immunol. 2020 May;52(3):121- 30.

13. Humaid AI, Ashraf AS, Masood KA, Nuha AS, Saleh DA, Awadh AM.

Prevalence and risk factors of otitis media with effusion in school children in Qassim region of Saudi Arabia. Int J Health Sci. 2014 Oct;8(4):325-34.

14. Saim A, Saim L, Saim S, Ruszymah BH, Sani A. Prevalence of otitis media with effusion amongst pre-school children in Malaysia. Int J Pediatr Otorhinolaryngol. 1997 Jul;41(1):21-8.
15. Malouche S, Boussetta K, Ben Hassine L, Malouche K, Siala M, Nessib F, et al. Skin sensitizations to pneumallergens in children: a cross-sectional study of 200 cases.Tunis Med. Oct 2013;91(11):627-32.
16. Annesi Maesano I, Didier A, Klossek M, Chanal I, Moreau D, Bousquet J. The score for allergic rhinitis (SFAR): a simple and valid assessment method in population studies. Allergy. 2002 Feb;57(2):107-14.
17. Umapathy D, Alles R, Scadding GK. A community based questionnaire study on the association between symptoms suggestive of otitis media with effusion, rhinitis and asthma in primary school children. Int J Pediatr Otorhinolaryngol. 2007 May;71(5):705-12.
18. Ciprandi G, Cirillo I, Vizzaccaro A, Tosca M, Passalacqua G, Pallestrini E, et al. Seasonal and perennial allergic rhinitis: is this classification adherent to real life? Allergy. 2005 Jul;60(7):882-7.
19. Roberts J, Hunter L, Gravel J, Rosenfeld R, Berman S, Haggard M, et al. Otitis media, hearing loss, and language learning: controversies and current research. J Dev Behav Pediatr. 2004 Apr;25(2):110-22.
20. Karli R, Balbaloglu E, Uzun L, Cinar F, Ugur MB. Correlation of symptoms with total IgE and specific IgE levels in patients presenting with allergic rhinitis. Ther Adv Respir Dis. 2013 Apr;7(2):75-9.
21. Bchir F, Chabbou A, Basly W, Guilloux L, Kamel A, Jeguirim MS, et al. The role of phadiatop in the screening of respiratory allergy. Arch Inst Pasteur Tunis. 1989 Jan;66(1-2):25-31
22. Mrassi H, Yangui F, Cherif H, Abdellatif S, Baya C, Triki M, et al. Clinical and allergenic particularities of respiratory allergy in Tunisian children. Rev Fr Allergol. Apr 2022;62(3):355.
23. Dayer E. Serum detection of allergen-specific IgE [Internet]. Rev Med Suisse. Oct 2005;1:1004-9.
24. Serrano E, Percodani J, Didier A. Allergic rhinitis. Rev Prat. 2000 Sep;50(14):1537-41.
25. Simpson SA, Lewis R, Van Der Voort J, Butler CC. Oral or topical nasal steroids for hearing loss associated with otitis media with effusion in children. Cochrane Database Syst Rev. 2011 May;(5):CD001935.

26. Roditi RE, Caradonna DS, Shin JJ. The proposed usage of intranasal steroids and antihistamines for otitis media with effusion. Curr Allergy Asthma Rep. 2019 Sep;19(10):47.

27. Mandel EM, Casselbrant ML. Antibiotics for otitis media with effusion. Minerva Pediatr. 2004 Oct;56(5):481-95.

28. Griffin G, Flynn CA. Antihistamines and/or decongestants for otitis media with effusion (OME) in children. Cochrane Database Syst Rev. 2011 Sep;2011(9):CD003423.

29. Simon F, Haggard M, Rosenfeld RM, Jia H, Peer S, Calmels MN, et al. International consensus (ICON) on management of otitis media with effusion in children. Eur Ann Otorhinolaryngol Head Neck Dis. 2018 Feb;135(1):33-9.

30. Pfaar O, Demoly P, Gerth Van Wijk R, Bonini S, Bousquet J, Canonica GW, et al. Recommendations for the standardization of clinical outcomes used in allergen immunotherapy trials for allergic rhinoconjunctivitis: an EAACI position paper. Allergy. 2014 Jul;69(7):854-67.

31. Daboussi S, Mhamdi S, Aichaouia C, Moetamri Z, Mejri I, Khadraoui M, et al. Sublingual allergen immunotherapy in Tunisia: safety and efficacy profile. Rev Fr Allergol. June 2018;58(4):299-303.

32. Nguyen LP, Manoukian JJ, Tewfik TL, Sobol SE, Joubert P, Mazer BD, et al. Evidence of allergic inflammation in the middle ear and nasopharynx in atopic children with otitis media with effusion. J Otolaryngol. 2004 Dec;33(6):345-51.

33. Hurst DS. Efficacy of allergy immunotherapy as a treatment for patients with chronic otitis media with effusion. Int J Pediatr Otorhinolaryngol. 2008 Aug;72(8):1215-23.

34. Hellström S, Groth A, Jörgensen F, Pettersson A, Ryding M, Uhlén I, et al. Ventilation tube treatment: a systematic review of the literature. Otolaryngol Head Neck Surg. 2011 Sep;145(3):383-95.

35. Vlastarakos PV, Nikolopoulos TP, Korres S, Tavoulari E, Tzagaroulakis A, Ferekidis E. Grommets in otitis media with effusion: the most frequent operation in children. But is it associated with significant complications? Eur J Pediatr. 2007 May;166(5):385-91.

36. Bjur KA, Lynch RL, Fenta YA, Yoo KH, Jacobson RM, Li X, et al. Assessment of the association between atopic conditions and tympanostomy tube placement in children. Allergy Asthma Proc. 2012 May;33(3):289-96.

37. Wan XM, Yang J. An analysis on the relationship between indwelling time after tube insertion and recurrence in children with secretory otitis media. Lin Chung Er Bi Yan Hou Tou Jing Wai Ke Za Zhi. 2017 Apr;31(7):500-3.

APPENDICES

Appendix 1: Data collection form

1. First name: Medical file number:
Age:
Gender:

2. Medical and surgical history:

• Recurrent AOM:

• Recurrent angina:

• Allergic disease: Allergic rhinitis/ Asthma/ Other:

• Other:

3. Environmental factors:

• Passive smoking:

• Humidity:

• Large family/ Community living:

• Crèche attendance:

• Breastfeeding: absent/ short duration/ sufficient duration

• Other:

4. Functional signs:

• Hearing loss:Earache:

• Academic delay:Language delay:

• Nasal pruritus:Nasal obstruction:

• Sneezing:Rhinorrhoea:

• Mouth breathing:

• Nocturnal swelling:

• Development time:

5. Physical examination:

- **General examination:**

- **Otological examination (otoscopy):**

Tympanum	Normal	Dull	Bubbles retro-tympanic	Pocket from shrinkage	Blue
Right ear					
Ear left					

• Rhinological examination:

■ Rhinoscopy:

• Normal

• Hypertrophy of the inferior turbinates

• Deviation of the nasal septum

■ Nasal endoscopy:

• Free Cavum

• Obstructive adenoid vegetation

• Non-obstructive adenoid vegetation

❖ Oropharyngeal examination:

• Eutrophic palatine tonsils

• Non-obstructive hypertrophic palatine tonsils

• Obstructive hypertrophic palatine tonsils

6. Paraclinical investigations:

❖ Initial audiometric assessment:

• Impedencemetry:

Tympanogram	Type A	Type B	Type C
Right ear			
Left ear			

• Pure tone audiometry:

Right ear (dB)	500Hz	1000Hz	2000Hz	4000Hz
Air conduction				
Bone conduction				
Right ear (dB)	500Hz	1000Hz	2000Hz	4000Hz
Air conduction				
Bone conduction				

- **Auditory evoked potentials:** YES / NO Result:
- **Speech and language assessment:**
- ❖ **Allergological assessment:**
- **Total IgE assay:** YES/ NO Rate=

- **Multi-allergenic test:** Positive/Negative

- **Allergenic skin test:** Positive/NegativeAllergens:

- **Specific IgE test:** Positive/NegativeAllergens:

7. Medical treatment:

- Antibiotic therapy:Molecule=/Posology=/Duration=

- Oral corticosteroid therapy:Molecule=/Posology=/Number of courses=
- Oral antihistamines:Molecule=/ Dosage=

- Nasal treatment: Saline/ Corticosteroids/ Suction derivatives
- Allergy immunotherapy: Allergen=

Channel= Duration=

8. Surgical treatment: placement of ATT:

- ❖ Indication:
- ❖ Surgical procedure performed under LA/GA:
- ❖ Type of ATT:
- ❖ Intraoperative incident(s):
- ❖ Post-operative follow-up:

9. Post-surgical evolution:

❖ **Check-up at one to three months post-operatively:**

• **Clinical results:**

- Functional signs:

- Otoscopic examination: TPA in place/ TPA migration/ Otorrhea

- Treatment received

• **Audiometric results:**

Right ear (dB)	500Hz	1000Hz	2000Hz	4000Hz
Air conduction				
Bone conduction				
Right ear (dB)	500Hz	1000Hz	2000Hz	4000Hz
Air conduction				
Bone conduction				

❖ **Six-month post-operative check-up:**

• **Clinical results:**

- Functional signs:

- Otoscopic examination: TPA in place/ TPA migration/ Otorrhea

- Treatment received

• **Audiometric results:**

Right ear (dB)	500Hz	1000Hz	2000Hz	4000Hz
Air conduction				
Bone conduction				
Right ear (dB)	500Hz	1000Hz	2000Hz	4000Hz
Air conduction				
Bone conduction				

❖ **Check after removal of the ATT:**

• **Duration of ATT installation:**

• **Clinical results:**

- Functional signs:

- Examination otoscopy: Perforation   perforation/ Atelectasis/ Cholesteatoma

• **Audiometric results:**

Right ear (dB)	500Hz	1000Hz	2000Hz	4000Hz
Air conduction				
Bone conduction				
Right ear (dB)	500Hz	1000Hz	2000Hz	4000Hz
Air conduction				
Bone conduction				

• **OSM strikes again:**

• **Post-operative setback:**

Appendix 2:ARIA classification of allergic rhinitis

(Allergic Rhinitis and its Impact on Asthma) Version 2017

Appendix 3: Tympanogram (Types of curves)

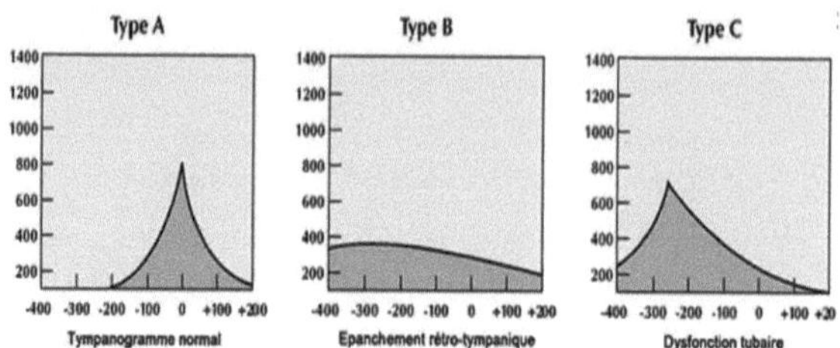

Appendix 4:Allergic rhinitis screening score: SFAR (Score for Allergic Rhinitis)

Score évaluant la probabilité qu'une rhinite chronique soit d'origine allergique	
Symptômes	**Points**
Obstruction nasale	1
Rhinorrhée	1
Prurit nasal/éternuements	1
Durée des symptômes	1 si > 6 mois 1 pour la saison pollinique (avril-juillet)
Association à une conjonctivite (larmoiement, rougeur, prurit)	2
Facteurs déclenchants : – épithélia d'animaux, moisissures – pollens, acariens, avec ou sans association aux précédents	 1 2
Réponse « oui » à la question : « Pensez-vous que votre enfant est allergique ? »	2
Dépistage positif d'allergie	2
Diagnostic positif d'allergie	1
Antécédents familiaux d'allergie	2

Nombre maximal de points : 16.
Un score < 7 n'est pas en faveur d'une rhinite allergique.

IMPACT OF ALLERGIC RHINITIS ON OPERATED OTITIS MEDIA WITH EFFUSION: CLINICAL, THERAPEUTIC AND AUDIOMETRIC ASPECTS
IN CHILDREN

Abstract

Introduction :

Otitis media with effusion (OME) represents the first cause of hearing loss and surgery in children. Allergic rhinitis (AR) has been identified as an independent risk factor for OME.

The objective of our study was to describe the impact of AR on clinical, therapeutic, and audiometric outcomes, in children undergoing surgery for OME.

Methods :

We conducted a monocentric retrospective study including school-aged children operated for OME with ventilation tube (VT) insertion at the department of otolaryngology of the military hospital of Tunis, during the period from 2014 to 2021. We compared the postoperative clinical and audiometric course of two groups of children (OME without AR and OME with AR).

Results :

We included 60 children with a mean age of 6.5 years. The mean hearing threshold was higher for the OME with AR group (43 dB versus 39.5 dB for the other group). The prevalence of AR was 43%. Dust mites were the most frequent allergens involved. The average hearing gain at three and six months after the insertion of the VT was lower for the OME with AR group (18 dB vs. 21.5 dB at three months and 16 dB vs. 18.5 dB at six months for the other group). The average duration of VT insertion was 13 months. After removal of the VT, the mean hearing threshold was 19 dB for the group OME without RA and 27 dB for the group OME with AR. Postoperatively, 32% of the children presented with otorrhea, of which 25% belonged to the group OME with AR. Recurrence of OME after removal of the VT was observed in 7% of the children (5% of the AR group and 2% of the non-AR group). The average postoperative follow-up was 17 months.

Conclusion:

AR represents an aggravating factor in OME-related hearing loss. Its early detection and treatment is essential in the management of OME in children.

Key words: Allergic rhinitis, Otitis media with effusion, Treatment, Evolution, Audiometry

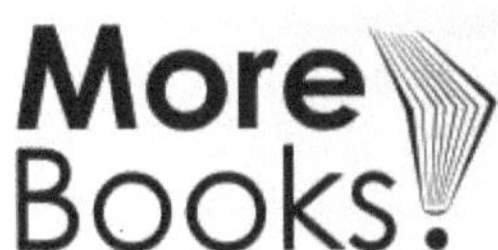

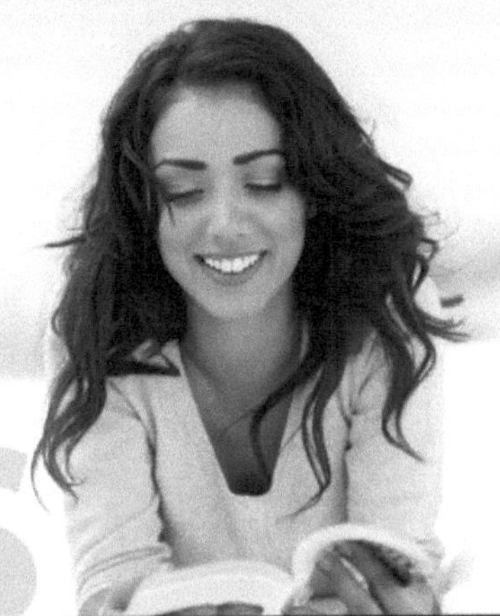

yes
I want morebooks!

Buy your books fast and straightforward online - at one of world's fastest growing online book stores! Environmentally sound due to Print-on-Demand technologies.

Buy your books online at
www.morebooks.shop

Kaufen Sie Ihre Bücher schnell und unkompliziert online – auf einer der am schnellsten wachsenden Buchhandelsplattformen weltweit! Dank Print-On-Demand umwelt- und ressourcenschonend produziert.

Bücher schneller online kaufen
www.morebooks.shop

info@omniscriptum.com
www.omniscriptum.com

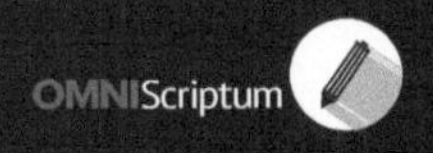

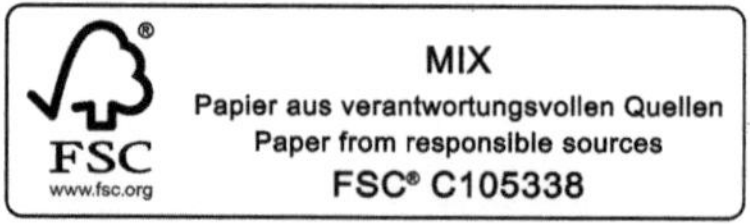

Printed by Books on Demand GmbH, Norderstedt / Germany